10-Day Green Smoothie Cleanse

Boost Vitality with the 10 day Green
Smoothie Cleanse

Rebecca Soto

Table of Contents

CHAPTER 4 – GREEN SMOOTHIE CLEANSE RECIPES TO ENJOY...22

Introduction

Are you ready to change your life? Have you decided it is time to take off those extra pounds and pursue a healthier lifestyle? Are you ready to lose weight, improve your health and start feeling amazing? If so, the green smoothie cleanse plan can help you jump-start your weight loss efforts. One of the main reasons that people have difficulty losing weight is because the body is full of toxins. Those toxins are stored in fat, and until you eliminate those toxins, it is difficult to burn off extra fat.

Since detoxifying is so important, going on the green smoothie detox is a great way to begin a new healthy lifestyle geared towards losing weight. As you follow the green smoothie diet, your body will begin eliminating all those toxins, preparing your body for weight loss. In fact, you will probably lose weight in the ten days that you follow the green smoothie cleanse. One of the green smoothie benefits is that you will be better able to eliminate old habits during your 10-day cleanse.

While a 10-day green smoothie cleanse may sound drastic, most people actually find that they enjoy the delicious green smoothie recipes they consume during the cleanse. In fact, you will probably enjoy your green smoothies so much that you'll want to continue enjoying the smoothies once a day after you complete the 10-day cleanse. Once you are done with the cleanse, it is a good idea to keep adding green smoothies to your diet, since they will help support weight loss and will help you make sure that you get all the nutrients that your body needs.

In this ebook, you will find everything you need to complete the 10-day green smoothie cleanse plan successfully. You will find helpful information on the green smoothie cleanse, a look at green smoothie benefits and tips for getting started with the cleanse. This recipe book is packed with green smoothie recipes, ensuring you have many different recipes to keep you from getting bored with your smoothies. You will also find a helpful 10-day eating plan that will help you plan your meals during the cleanse. With this book to guide you, you can start the cleanse and get on your way to a healthier body.

Chapter 1 – What is a Green Smoothie Cleanse?

What is the green smoothie cleanse? It's a detox cleanse that lasts for ten days and involves drinking green smoothies for every meal. The green smoothies all include green leafy veggies, but they can have water, fruits and other veggies added to them as well. While you may think that you will feel hungry all the time, since you are only drinking smoothies, you actually will find that the smoothies fill you up and provide you with all the nutrients your body needs. Most people actually notice that they have more energy and they feel great while on the 10-day green smoothie cleanse plan.

The Importance of Detoxifying Your Body

If your primary goal is to lose weight and embark on a healthier lifestyle, you may wonder why you should kick start your weight loss efforts with a green smoothie detox. Will this program really help you to lose those extra pounds when other diets have not work? Yes!

Unfortunately, we are exposed to many toxins in the environment and the foods we eat. Those toxins built up in the body and can result in weight gain over time. If the toxin load because too heavy for the body, the body puts all its energy into trying to eliminate toxins instead of working on burning calories. This means that your body no longer has the energy to burn fat. Once you eliminate those toxins, the body can go back to burning fat instead of having to focus all its energy on flushing out toxins.

Many people try diets to lose weight and get discouraged when they don't see the results they want. This occurs because most diets fail to address all the toxins in the body. Just a few of the signs that your body may be dealing with too many toxins include weight gain, fatigue, constipation, headaches, digestion issues, bloating and low levels of energy.

The green smoothie diet works differently from other diets. It immediately starts working to detoxify your body. Through the 10 days you are on the cleanse, your body will begin eliminating all the toxins that have built up in your body. As the toxins are eliminated, most people see some initial weight loss. Once you finish the cleanse, your body will be primed and ready for optimal weight loss, since you will have eliminated the toxins stored in your body. This diet sets you up for weight loss success.

Is the Cleanse Right for You?

You may be wondering if the green smoothie cleanse plan is right for you. How do you know if your body has built up toxins? Here are a few of the signs that the green smoothie detox is a great choice for you:

- You are a smoker or you live with a smoker

- You find it difficult to sleep

- You're not getting enough sleep each night

- You constantly crave sweets

- You deal with yeast infections regularly

- You consume meats, veggies and fruits that are not organic

- You live in an urban area

- You take medications, such as antidepressants or antibiotics

- You don't drink enough water daily

- You regularly consume processed foods

- You get sick often

- You deal with skin problems, such as rashes or acne

- You feel fatigued and tired all the time

- You use beauty products and household products that contain chemicals

If you identify with more than one of these signs, there is a good chance that your body is dealing with toxin overload. This means that the green smoothie cleanse is an excellent choice for you and should offer you great results.

How the Cleanse Works

Now that you know that the green smoothie detox is right for you, you may be wondering how the cleanse works. The cleanse lasts for ten days. During those ten days, you should be drinking green smoothies throughout the day. It's recommended that you consume up to 60 ounces of the smoothies each day for the best results. You can prepare the smoothies at meal times or prepare them in the morning so you can just sip on them throughout your day.

Along with the green smoothies, you need to drink plenty of water. You should have a minimum of 64 ounces of water each day. Herbal and detox teas, such as green tea, count as part of your water intake. While it is okay to have some small snacks throughout the day if you need them, you need to avoid eating or drinking certain foods, such as processed foods, refined carbs, foods with refined sugar, meats, alcoholic beverages, milk products and fried foods. Small snacks that are okay include raw seeds or nuts, crunchy veggies like cucumbers, celery or carrots, or some apples.

Chapter 2 – Benefits of a Green Smoothie Cleanse

Going on a green smoothie cleanse offers many wonderful benefits. When you follow the green smoothie diet, you will soon begin to notice some benefits, such as weight loss, improved energy and more. In fact, drinking green smoothies offer so many benefits that you will probably want to continue adding them to your diet, even after you complete the cleanse. Here are just a few benefits that following the green smoothie cleanse plan can offer you.

Benefit #1 – Jump Starts Weight Loss

One of the main benefits of going on a green smoothie detox is that it helps to jump start weight loss. Even though the smoothies fill you up, the smoothies will help you lose weight. Since the smoothies have a high water content and they are packed with low calorie green leafy veggies, they'll help you take off those extra pounds. They are low in calories, yet they have plenty of fiber in them, which will make you feel full. Because the fiber makes you feel full, drinking the smoothies will help eliminate cravings, which will aid in weight loss as well.

Benefit #2 – Increase Intake of Important Nutrients

Another benefit of going on the green smoothie cleanse is that the smoothies help to increase your intake of important nutrients. Since the veggies and fruits in the smoothies are raw, they offer you more nutrients than cooked fruits and veggies do. The green smoothies you drink on this diet are packed with important antioxidants, vitamins, fiber, phytonutrients, minerals and more. Your body needs the nutrients found in the smoothies. Unfortunately, many people do not get the nutrients they need from their diet. However, when fruits and veggies are turned into smoothies, it makes it easier to get more fruits and veggies in your diet, improving your intake of the important nutrients that your body needs to function optimally.

Benefit #3 – Look and Feel Young and Healthy

You may be surprised that consuming green smoothies offers the benefit of helping you look and feel young and healthy. All the nutrients found in the raw fruits and veggies improve the function of your body and help to improve the health of your body. As you eliminate toxins from the body, you will notice that your skin begins to improve, looking younger and healthier. The skin is the body's largest organ and all those toxins can negatively affect skin. As you remove the toxins, you can expect skin to improve. All the antioxidants in the green smoothies will also help to reverse and prevent aging, reducing problems with fine lines, age spots and wrinkles, giving you a more youthful appearance. Not only will you look young and healthy, but the improvement in your body's functions will make you feel younger and healthier as well.

Benefit #4 – Eliminate Toxins from the Body

The body is designed to eliminate toxins naturally. However, when excessive toxins build up in the body, the body may have a tough time keeping up with all the toxins. To reduce the strain of your body, you can take measures to help your body eliminate those toxins. The green smoothie cleanse helps the body as it works to eliminate toxins. All the fiber in the green smoothies help the body to cleanse away built up waste and toxins. This helps reduce the strain of the toxic load on your body and as toxins are eliminating, you'll notice that you begin feeling better. In fact, many of the symptoms of a high toxic load, such as headaches, fatigue and constipation, will go away once those toxins are eliminated.

Benefit #5 – Hydrate the Body for Improved Bodily Functions

Many people today walk around consistently dehydrated. Since most functions in the body rely on water, dehydration can result in big problems. When your body is well hydrated, it ensures that the immune system, brain, digestive system, muscles and other functions all work the way they should. Regularly smoking, eating processed foods or consuming sodas may result in dehydration. Check your urine if you want to know if you're dehydrated. If it's not clean or a very pale yellow, then you probably are dealing with dehydration. Since green smoothies have such a high water content, they help to rehydrate the body, which improves all bodily functions. Drinking the smoothies is a tasty way to get more water in your diet as well.

Benefit #6 – Improves Performance of the Digestive System

Following the green smoothie cleanse plan will also help improve the performance of your digestive system. Since the smoothies are in liquid form, the body can easily metabolize and digest them, making it easier for the body to get the nutrients it needs from those fruits and veggies. If you are dealing with digestive problems, such as irritable bowel syndrome, acid reflux, heartburn or colitis, you may find that drinking green smoothies helps treat these problems. Eating fried foods, too much gluten and processed foods can lead to digestive problems, as can consuming a large amount of unhealthy fats. The digestive system doesn't need to work hard to digest green smoothies, since they are already in liquid form. This helps take some of the pressure off the digestive system and makes it easy for your body to extract all the important nutrients that your body needs to function optimally.

Benefit #7 – Tasty, Easy Options to Try

Many people find that they love the green smoothie diet because there are so many tasty, easy options to try. Preparing the smoothies is a breeze and most smoothies only take a few minutes to prepare. Easy preparation makes it easy for you to stick to this diet. Of course, all the tasty green smoothie recipes are beneficial as well. Since most of the green smoothie recipes include fruits, the included fruits will shine through so you won't really end up tasting the greens. With so many tasty greens and delicious fruits and veggies available, you will find so many delicious recipes to try. In fact, you can even start experimenting with your own recipes. You definitely won't get tired of green smoothies, since there are so many different options available to you.

Chapter 3 – Getting Started with the Green Smoothie Cleanse

To ensure that you are successful when you start the green smoothie diet, you'll need to learn about the greens you should use, fruits and veggies that are acceptable in your smoothies and foods you should avoid while you are following the green smoothie cleanse. If your health or your lifestyle keeps you from following a complete 10-day cleanse, you can also learn how to do a modified cleanse, which will still offer you many of the benefits that come with a green smoothie detox.

Greens to Use in Your Green Smoothies

Greens are the essential ingredient in your green smoothies, since they are packed with important nutrients, fiber and water. When following the green smoothie cleanse, it's a good idea to vary the greens you use in your smoothies from time to time to ensure you get a wider variety of nutrients. Here are some of the best greens you can use in your green smoothie recipes.

- **Spinach** – Spinach is one of the most well-known and well-liked dark leafy green veggies. It's also the most popular green veggie used in many green smoothie recipes. Spinach has a very mild taste, which is why it is such a great ingredient to use in your smoothies. It offers many nutrients, including vitamins K, A, E and C, as well as magnesium, omega-3 fatty acids and calcium.

- **Kale** – Kale, another popular green leafy veggie, tastes wonderful in smoothies as well. The delicate ruffled leaves are packed with vitamin K, C and A. Studies show that kale may help to reduce the risk of certain types of cancers.

- **Arugula** – The peppery, zippy arugula leaves are excellent for brain and bone healthy. Arugula offers important nutrients, including vitamins K, C, A and folic acid.

- **Lettuce** – Many types of lettuce exist and for your green smoothies, it's best to choose dark green lettuce leaves. Romaine lettuce is the most popular type of lettuce used for the green smoothie diet, since it contains folic acid and vitamins K, A and C.

- **Chard** – Chard has a nice texture and tastes a bit like beets. It is an excellent choice in green smoothies because it helps to clean out your digestive system and studies show it may help prevent certain types of cancer.

- **Turnip Greens –** While turnip greens have plenty of flavor, they have a bitter taste, so you will want to pair them with some sweet fruits to counteract the bitter taste. However, they offer great healthy benefits, including helping to fight cancer.

- **Beet Greens –** Studies show that beet greens help to give the immune system a boost, improve vision and prevent Alzheimer's disease. They are also an excellent source of vitamin K.

- **Parsley –** Many people think of parsley as a garnish, but it packs a great nutritional punch too. It is packed with plenty of fiber, minerals, vitamins and antioxidants. The antioxidants fight the signs of aging and studies show that parsley does an excellent job at keeping blood sugar levels stable.

- **Bok Choy –** Bok Choy is crunch and has a very milk taste. The antioxidants, calcium and vitamin content make it an excellent addition to your smoothies.

Other Foods to Include in Your Smoothies

While green leafy veggies are the base of your green smoothies, you can include many other foods in your smoothies as well. Adding other foods can help you to improve the flavor and you can add in foods that will add to the nutrient content of your smoothies as well. Here is a look at other foods you can add to smoothies to improve taste and their nutritional punch.

- **Fruits** – Fruits help to improve the taste of your green smoothies and can be added to your smoothies. However, you shouldn't overdo the fruits. Diabetics should make sure they choose low sugar fruits. Many of the best green smoothie recipes call for various fruits, which also pack in many important nutrients for your body. Fruits to add to your smoothies include, but are not limited to, the following:

Pineapple

Mango

Blueberries

Apples

Raspberries

Strawberries

Bananas

Lemons

Cherries

Limes

Cranberries

Kiwi

Papaya

Grapes

Peaches

- **Sweeteners** – Natural sweeteners can be added to green smoothies if necessary, but it's best to leave them out if possible. Sweeteners like Stevia, organic maple syrup or agave are okay.

- **Water** – Purified water can be added to smoothies. It helps improve hydration and can be used to thin out the texture of your smoothies. Using purified or spring water is important, since you want to avoid using water that may have chemicals in it.

- **Protein** – Consider adding protein to your green smoothies, especially if you are working out or need some extra energy to your day. It is best to avoid whey protein powder. Instead, go with hemp protein, soy protein or rice protein powders. Adding protein to your smoothies is especially important if you are planning to work out after drinking your smoothie. You may even want to add protein to smoothies to help kick start a busy day.

- **Veggies** – You can also add other veggies to your smoothies. Tasty veggies to add include the following:

Cucumbers

Tomatoes

Carrots

Zucchini

Celery

And other favorite veggies

Foods to Avoid While on the Green Smoothie Cleanse

Certain foods should be avoided while you are following the green smoothie diet. Keep a list of the foods you should avoid so you don't accidentally consume them while you're on the cleanse. Foods you should avoid include the following:

- Starchy veggies, such as corn and potatoes

- Refined carbs (donuts, white pastas, white bread)

- Meat

- Dairy products (cheese, milk, yogurt, ice cream)

- Sodas

- Refined sugar

- Alcoholic beverages

- Anything fried

- Unhealthy fats

- Coffee

- Processed foods

About a Modified Cleanse

Some people may not be able to handle the full 10-day green smoothie cleanse, particularly those with certain health problems. However, you can do a modified cleanse that will allow you to enjoy the benefits of the cleanse.

To do a modified cleanse, you will need to drink smoothies for breakfast and lunch and then you can have a light, healthy meal for dinner. Drink 4-5 16oz green smoothies throughout the day. Then, for dinner, choose a healthy option, such as grilled fish with broccoli and a side salad. Small snacks are okay on a modified cleanse as well, as long as you make healthy choice.

Of course, if you do a modified cleanse, you still need to skip foods on the list of foods to avoid. Drinking water is important as well.

Chapter 4 – Green Smoothie Cleanse Recipes to Enjoy

Now that you have learned more about the green smoothie diet and how to get started, it's time to start making your green smoothies. While you can always make your own smoothie recipes, we have provide you with a large selection of green smoothie recipes to get you started. You will find a huge selection of different flavors, whether you want something spicy, something sweet or something packed with a bit of extra protein. As you embark on your green smoothie cleanse, use these recipes for healthy, delicious smoothies. Once you try several of our recipes, you may be inspired to come up with a few great recipes of your own.

Cherry, Blueberry and Raspberry Green Smoothie Recipe

This smoothie combines raspberries, blueberries and cherries for a tasty green breakfast smoothie. Not only does it taste amazing, but the combination of berries and cherries ensure you get a great dose of vitamin C, fiber and important antioxidants that help fight off disease. Once you taste this smoothie, you will definitely want to make this one again.

What You'll Need:

- 2 cups of purified water

- 1 banana

- 2 cups of fresh spinach leaves

- ½ cup of blueberries

- ½ cup of raspberries

- 1 cup of cherries, pits removed

How to Make It:

Wash all the berries, cherries and spinach before using. Remove pits from the cherries. Cut the banana into chunks. Add the water and the spinach to your blender. Blend until the mixture is smooth. Add the chunks of banana and continue blending. Last, place berries in the blender and continue to blend until you have a smooth mixture. Pour smoothie two glasses and enjoy. You can drink the second glass later in the day if desired.

NOTE: Use frozen berries for a cold, refreshing smoothie.

Grapefruit and Kale Green Smoothie Recipe

If you enjoy tart flavors, such as grapefruit, you will enjoy this tasty grapefruit and kale green smoothie. The lime, tart green apple and grapefruit offer a nice, tart kick, making this a perfect smoothie to drink in the morning when you need something to perk you up.

What You'll Need:

- ½ cucumber, sliced

- 1 medium Granny Smith apple

- 4 stalks of celery

- 1 grapefruit, peel removed

- 1 lime, peel removed

- 1 head of kale, stems removed

- 1 cup of water

How to Make It:

Core and peel the apple and remove the peel from the grapefruit and lime. Cut the apple into chunks. Place the kale leaves, cucumber slices and the water in your blender, blending until smooth. Add the celery and blend again. Add the apple pieces, grapefruit and lime to the blender. Continue blending until you have a smooth mixture. You can add more purified water if the smoothie is too thick.

Pina Colada Flavored Spinach and Almond Milk Green Smoothie Recipe

You are not supposed to have alcohol while on the green smoothie cleanse. However, if you love pina coladas, this smoothie, inspired by a recipe by GreenSmoothies.com will allow you to enjoy all those delicious flavors without all the calories that come with alcohol. If you start craving something sweet, try this green smoothie, since it is sure to eliminate your cravings for sweets.

What You'll Need:

- 3 cups of fresh pineapple, chunked

- 2 cups of fresh spinach leaves

- 2 tablespoons of unsweetened coconut flakes

- ½ cup of coconut water

- 1.5 cups of unsweetened almond milk

How to Make It:

Wash the spinach and use a salad spinner to spin it dry. Cut pineapple into chunks.

Add the coconut water, almond milk and spinach to your blender. Blend until the spinach and liquids form a smooth mixture. Add the coconut flakes and the pineapple, blending once again until the mixture reaches the desired consistency. Sprinkle a few coconut flakes on top for a nice topping. Makes two servings.

Sweet Blueberry and Romaine Green Smoothie Recipe

Blueberries are packed with healthy antioxidants and romaine lettuce offers many excellent nutrients as well. This recipe combines crisp romaine with sweet blueberries and it's a winning combination. The addition of the apple adds more fiber and the lime gives the green smoothie a nice zip.

What You'll Need:

- ¾ cup of frozen blueberries

- 2 cups of purified water

- 1 green apple, chopped

- 1 head of romaine lettuce

- ¼ lime, peeled

How to Make It:

Wash the apple and then chop it into chunks. Wash the romaine lettuce and dry thoroughly. Peel the rind off the piece of lime.

Add the water to the blender and then place the romaine lettuce in the blender. Blend until the lettuce and water make a smoothie, liquid mixture. Add the lime, apple chunks and the frozen blueberries and continue to blend. Blend until the smoothie reaches your preferred consistency. Add more water if needed to thin the mixture.

Grape, Peach and Coconut Green Smoothie Recipe

This yummy combination of coconut water, peaches and grapes makes two servings, so enjoy one as a green breakfast smoothie and enjoy the second serving later for an afternoon pick me up. If desired, you can add a banana to increase the potassium content while adding some extra sweetness.

What You'll Need:

- 2 peaches, peeled and pits removed

- 2 cups of fresh spinach

- 2 cups of green grapes

- 1 cup of coconut water

How to Make It:

Wash the peaches and then peel them and remove the pits. Wash the grapes and spinach as well. Remove any stems from the spinach. Place the coconut water and fresh spinach in the blender, blending until the mixture becomes smooth. Add grapes and peaches and keep blending. If needed, add a bit more coconut water. You can also add a few ice cubes to make the smoothie cold and refreshing. Makes two servings.

Tropical Fruit and Green Leaf Lettuce Green Smoothie Recipe

Do you like tropical fruit? If so, you are going to love the flavor explosion this green smoothie provides. The banana helps to make the smoothie smoother and offers great nutrients. The pineapple combines with the banana to make a delicious, tropical flavor. You will enjoy all the nutrients that come from the green leaf lettuce, but you probably will barely know the lettuce is there, since the tropical flavors are so prevalent.

What You'll Need:

- 1 large banana

- 1 head of green leaf lettuce

- ½ of a fresh pineapple

- 2 cups of purified water

How to Make It:

Peel the banana and then cut it into chunks. Wash the green leaf lettuce thoroughly. Remove the core and skin from the pineapple. Cut half of it into chunks and store the rest of the pineapple in the refrigerator to use in another green smoothie recipe.

Place the green leaf lettuce and water in your blending.

Blend on high until the mixture becomes smooth. Place the banana chunks and pineapple chunks in the blender, continuing to blend until your smoothie reaches your desired consistency. Enjoy right away.

Pomegranate, Orange and Banana Green Smoothie Recipe

Pomegranate is such a delicious, healthy fruit, but many people rarely eat pomegranate seeds. The pomegranate seeds turn this smoothie into something special and the addition of orange juice packs in even more vitamin C, which boosts your immune system. The combination of flavors is delicious and you will get plenty of antioxidants when you drink this smoothie as part of your green smoothie cleanse.

What You'll Need:

- 1 ¼ cups of purified water

- 1 banana

- ¾ cup of orange juice (preferably freshly squeezed orange juice)

- 1 cup of pomegranate seeds

- 2 cups of fresh spinach

How to Make It:

Peel the banana and wash the spinach. Remove the pomegranate seeds from the pomegranate.

Add the purified water, orange juice and spinach to your

blender. Process until you have a thick, smooth mixture. Add the banana in chunks to the blender and then place the pomegranate seeds in the blender as well. Continue blending until your smoothie is finished. You can thin it if needed with a little more orange juice or water. Makes two servings.

Spicy Cilantro and Romaine Green Smoothie Recipe

While many of the green smoothie recipes call for fruit, adding sweetness to the smoothies, this smoothie is actually spicy and only includes veggies. If you want something different that has a nice, spicy kick, this is the smoothie for you. The jalapeno, cilantro and ginger all combine to make a flavorful drink that you are sure to enjoy.

What You'll Need:

- 1 cucumber

- ½ lemon, peel removed

- ½ head of romaine lettuce

- 2 celery stalks

- 1 clove of garlic, peeled and chopped

- ½ head of cilantro

- ½ onion

- ½ jalapeno, step and seeds removed

- 1 inch piece of fresh ginger

- 1 cup of water

How to Make It:

Wash all of the vegetables before making your smoothie. Cut the cucumber, celery stalks, onion and ginger into chunks. Chop the jalapeno and garlic too. Make sure that the peel is removed from the lemon you are using.

Add the water, cilantro and romaine lettuce to your blender. Blend until combined and smooth. Add the lemon, celery, cucumber, garlic, onion, jalapeno and ginger. Continue blending. Add more water if the mixture is too thick. Blend until mixture reaches your desired consistency. Makes two servings.

Romaine and Banana Green Smoothie Recipe

Bananas are always a wonderful addition to green smoothies and this smoothie combines romaine lettuce and bananas. The parsley, cilantro and apples kick up the flavor too and add important nutrients that your body needs to the green smoothie.

What You'll Need:

- 1 banana, chunked

- 1 ½ cups of cold water

- 1/3 bunch of fresh parsley

- 1 head of romaine lettuce, chopped

- ½ fresh lemon, juiced

- 3 stalks of celery

- 1/3 bunch of fresh cilantro

- 2 green apples

How to Make It:

Peel the banana. Wash the romaine, parsley and cilantro. Cut the celery into chunks. Juice the ½ lemon and reserve juice. Wash the apple and then remove the core. Chop the apple into pieces.

In the blender, combine the chopped romaine lettuce, parsley, cilantro and water. Blend on low until the mixture becomes smooth. Next, add the apples and celery to the mixture, increasing the blending speed. Last, add the lemon juice and banana chunks, continuing to blend until the entire mixture is smooth. Enjoy right away. Makes 4 servings.

Berry, Kiwi and Avocado Green Smoothie Recipe

The berries used in this smoothie recipe are full of wonderful antioxidants, which help to fight free radicals, preventing cancer, aging and more. The kiwi adds even more vitamin C to the smoothie, and the spinach is packed with nutrients, such as iron. You may be surprised to see the addition of avocado to this smoothie, but it adds healthy fats and gives the smoothie a nice texture as well.

What You'll Need:

- 1 kiwi, chopped

- 2 cups of purified water

- ½ avocado, chopped

- 1 cup of blueberries

- 1 cup of frozen raspberries or strawberries

- 2 cups of fresh spinach, stems removed

- 1 banana, chunked

How to Make It:

Wash the spinach and the blueberries. Peel the banana and then chop into big chunks. Cut an avocado in half, use the side that doesn't have the seed and chunk the avocado. Wash and then chop the kiwi.

Blend the spinach and the water together in your blender. Once the mixture becomes nice and smooth, add the kiwi, avocado, blueberries, frozen raspberries and banana chunks to the blender. Continue blending until the mixture is well blended. Makes two delicious servings.

Peach and Spinach Green Smoothie Recipe

This recipe is inspired by a recipe from DrBenKim.com and combines the goodness of peaches, orange juice and spinach together. It is a very simple green smoothie recipe that requires very little time to make. If you enjoy peaches, you are sure to tempt your taste buds while providing you with plenty of essential nutrients.

What You'll Need:

- ½ cup of cold, purified water

- 2 cups of fresh spinach leaves

- 1 cup of fresh squeezed orange juice

- 2 peaches

How to Make It:

Wash the spinach leaves and set to the side to dry. Squeeze your orange juice. Wash peaches. Peel the peaches and remove the pit. Chop the peaches into pieces.

In the blender, blend together the water, orange juice and the spinach leaves. Once the mixture is smooth, add the peach pieces to the blender. Keep blending until you have a thick, smooth consistency. If the mixture is too thick, add a little more orange juice or some water.

Baby Lettuce and Pineapple Green Smoothie Recipe

For this green smoothie you can use your favorite baby lettuces along with some kale. The pineapple provides sweetness to the smoothie and the banana gives the smoothie a nice texture. Since this recipe only makes a single serving, you may want to double the recipe.

What You'll Need:

- ½ of a banana, cut into chunks

- 1 cup of purified water, cold

- 1 cup of raw kale, chopped

- 1 cup of baby lettuces

- ¼ cup of pineapple, fresh

- ¼ cup of parsley, fresh

How to Make It:

Peel a banana and chunk half of it for the smoothie. Wash kale and then chop it into pieces. Chop the pineapple into chunks. Wash the parsley and baby lettuces.

Add the water, kale, baby lettuces and parsley to your blender. Blend on low until the greens combine with the water, creating a smooth mixture. Next, add the banana and pineapple chunks to your blender. Increase the speed and continue blending. Once you have a smooth texture, pour the smoothie in a glass and enjoy. Makes one serving.

Almond Butter and Sweet Red Grape Green Smoothie Recipe

If you enjoy the combined flavors of peanut butter and jelly, this smoothie will take you back to your childhood. Inspired by a recipe from Greensmoothies.com, it combines almond butter with yummy red grapes, giving it that peanut butter and jelly flavor. The almond butter tastes wonderful and adds some protein and healthy fats to your smoothie. The grapes and spinach include important phytonutrients and antioxidants. The almond milk and bananas gives this delicious green smoothie recipe a creamy, smooth texture.

What You'll Need:

- 2 cups of sweet red grapes

- 4 tablespoons of almond butter

- 2 cups of fresh baby spinach leaves

- 2 bananas

- 2 cups of unsweetened almond milk

How to Make It:

Wash the red grapes and the baby spinach. Peel the bananas and then cut them into chunks.

Place the almond milk in the blender and then add the spinach. Start blending on low until the mixture is smooth. Add the grapes, bananas and the almond butter. Keep blending, increasing the speed. Continue until the mixture is thick and creamy. Makes two servings.

NOTE: Try freezing the grapes several hours before making this green smoothie, which will result in a cold, refreshing smoothie.

Mango, Banana and Spinach Green Smoothie Recipe

Mangos pack a powerful punch of important nutrients and bananas pack in potassium and other nutrients. This smoothie combines the flavor of bananas and mangos, which results in a flavorful drink. While the recipe calls for spinach, you could always substitute in other mild dark leafy greens if you want.

What You'll Need:

2 large mangos

1 medium banana

2 cups of fresh spinach leaves

1 cup of purified water

How to Make It:

Peel the mangos and then chop them into medium sized pieces. Peel the banana and chop. Wash the spinach before using it in your smoothie.

Place the cup of water and the fresh spinach leaves in your blender, blending on low until smooth and well combined. Add the pieces of banana and mango to the mixture. Increase blender speed and keep blending until the mixture reaches smoothie consistency. Add a little water if the mixture becomes too thick. Makes 1 serving. Enjoy!

Protein Powder and Chia Seed Green Smoothie Recipe

When you need a powerful protein punch, you will want to whip up this protein powder and chia seed green smoothie recipe. Just make sure that you are using the right protein powder – you should not be using a whey protein powder while you are following the green smoothie cleanse, since whey protein powder has dairy in it. Instead, go with a hemp or soy protein powder when making this smoothie. This smoothie is not as sweet as some of the others, but it will give you the protein you need, whether you are working out or you have a long, tough day ahead of you.

What You'll Need:

- 2 bananas

- 2 cups of coconut water

- 3 cups of fresh spinach leaves

- 1 scoop of soy or hemp protein powder

- 1 tablespoon of chia seeds

How to Make It:

Peel and chop the bananas. Wash spinach leaves thoroughly.

In the blender, blend together the coconut water and the spinach leaves until your mixture is creamy and smooth. Add the banana chunks, protein powder and chia seeds to the mixture. Continue blending until your mixture turns into a smooth, creamy drink. Pour into a glass and top with a few more chia seeds if desired. Makes one serving.

Coconut, Almond and Cantaloupe Green Smoothie Recipe

The cantaloupe in this green smoothie offers folate, vitamin C, potassium, carotenoids and other important nutrients. Coconut oil is also included in the smoothie, which offers your body some healthy fats, which are important for heart health. The combination of the coconut oil, cantaloupe and grapes offers a light, delicious flavor.

What You'll Need:

- ½ of a fresh cantaloupe, rind removed

- 2 cups of fresh spinach leaves

- 2 tablespoons of coconut oil

- ½ cup of water

- 1 cup of red grapes

- 1 cup of unsweetened almond milk

How to Make It:

Remove the rind from the cantaloupe and cut ½ of it into chunks. Store the other half for another smoothie or enjoy it as a snack later. Wash spinach leaves thoroughly. Wash red grapes before using.

Add the almond milk, coconut oil, water and spinach leaves to your blender. Begin blending on low, continuing until your mixture becomes smooth. Place the cantaloupe pieces and grapes in the blender and continue blending. Increase blender speed if necessary and keep blending until you get the consistency you want from the smoothie. Makes two servings. Enjoy immediately.

Romaine, Strawberry and Grape Green Smoothie Recipe

For this smoothie, you will want to use frozen strawberries, which will result in a cold, delicious smoothie that is perfect for a warm day. You can also freeze the banana called for, but if you do this, make sure you freeze the banana in chunks so it is easier to blend. When the weather is hot, you will want to whip up this smoothie several times a day to beat the heat. In fact, it continues to be a great, refreshing drink, even after you finish the green smoothie cleanse plan.

What You'll Need:

- 1 banana, chopped and frozen

- 1 cup of red grapes, seedless

- 1 cup of frozen strawberries

- ½ head of fresh romaine lettuce

How to Make It:

Take the time to wash the grapes and the romaine lettuce. Make sure you peel and chop the banana ahead of time, placing the chunks in the freezer for a few hours.

Place the grapes in the bottom of the blender. Blend

until the grapes start creating a liquid. Add the romaine lettuce and continue blending. If needed, add a little water so you end up with a smooth mixture of grapes and lettuce. Add the frozen strawberries and frozen banana pieces. Continue blending until you have a cold, thick smoothie. Add more water as needed. Makes 1 big serving, so double if you are serving more than one person. Enjoy while cold.

Mango, Pineapple and Cilantro Green Smoothie Recipe

You probably wouldn't think about combining cilantro with mango and pineapple, but the herb really adds a unique flavor with the tasty fruits. The avocado adds healthy fats and makes the smoothie a bit smoother and silkier. If desired, you can substitute in coconut water for the purified water, adding another layer of flavor to this delicious green smoothie.

What You'll Need:

- ½ of a ripe avocado

- ½ cup of fresh cilantro

- 1 cup of frozen pineapple chunks

- 1 ½ cups of fresh spinach

- 2 cups of water

- 1 ½ cups of fresh mango, chopped

How to Make It:

Wash the cilantro and the spinach. Remove the peel from the mango and then chop into large pieces.

Place the cilantro, spinach and water in your blender. Start blending on low and continue until the mixture is thick and smooth. Add the avocado, pineapple chunks and mango chunks to the spinach mixture. Continue blending, increasing the blender speed if necessary. Allow to blend until the mixture is smooth and thick. Pour into two glasses. Enjoy while cool. Makes two servings.

Flaxseed Berry Blend Green Smoothie Recipe

If you want a green breakfast smoothie that does not require work in the morning, try this one. You can make it the night before and store it in the refrigerator overnight. This way you can grab it on your way out the door and you do not have to worry about finding the time to make a delicious smoothie. It is packed with fruits that contain important vitamins and minerals for your body. The raw protein vegan water gives it a nice protein kick for your day and the spinach is the green part of the smoothie.

What You'll Need:

- 2 cups of fresh spinach leaves

- 1 green apple, chopped

- ½ cup of red seedless grapes

- ½ cup of chopped mango

- 1 cup of frozen strawberries

- 1 cup of raw protein vegan water

- 2 tablespoons of flaxseed

- 1 teaspoon of stevia (if desired)

How to Make It:

Wash the apple, grapes, mango and spinach leaves. Core the apple and chop it into pieces. Remove the peel from the mango and then chop into pieces.

Place the raw protein vegan water, the flaxseed and the spinach leaves into your blender and start blending on low. Once the mixture is smooth, add in the apple chunks, grapes, mango chunks, frozen strawberries and stevia (if desired). Keep blending, increasing the blender speed until your mixture is nice and smooth. Taste and add more stevia if you think it needs more sweetness. Makes two servings. Refrigerate and enjoy for breakfast.

Pear, Apple and Banana Green Smoothie Recipe

Pears, apples and bananas come together in this wonderful green smoothie recipe inspired by a recipe from KimberlySnyder.net. Along with the sweet fruits, the smoothie includes celery, cilantro, romaine lettuce, spinach and parsley. The best part about this smoothie is that the green smoothie recipes makes a huge batch, so you can make this in the morning and drink on it all day long. All the nutrients in this smoothie will make you feel great and will help you detox while you are on the green smoothie cleanse.

What You'll Need:

- 1 banana

- 2 cups of fresh spinach leaves

- ½ bunch of cilantro

- ½ bunch of parsley

- 1 head of romaine lettuce

- ½ lemon

- 4 stalks of celery

- 1 pear

- 1 apple

- 2 cups of purified water

How to Make It:

Wash the spinach, romaine, celery, parsley and cilantro. Chop the romaine lettuce and cut the celery into chunks. Wash the pear and the apple. Remove their cores and then cut into chunks. Peel and chunk the banana. Peel the lemon and remove any seeds.

Add the celery, romaine, cilantro, parsley, spinach and water all in your blender, putting the water at the very bottom of the blender. Turn on the slowest speed and begin blending. Increase speed as needed to turn the ingredients into a smooth liquid. Once smooth, remove the lid and add the lemon, banana chunks, pear chunks and apple chunks to the blender. Start on slow again and then begin increasing the speed until the speed is on high. Keep blending until the smoothie reaches the consistency you desire.

Makes 5 12-ounce servings. Enjoy one serving and save the rest for later in the day, making sure you refrigerate the servings you do not drink right away.

Ginger Cilantro Limeade Green Smoothie Recipe

The lime in this green smoothie is really refreshing, especially when added to the flavors of ginger and cilantro. You can have this smoothie ready in a jiffy, since it's one of the easier recipes out there. The bananas pack in a lot of fiber and potassium.

What You'll Need:

- 2 cups of purified water

- 1 lime

- 1 ½ cups of fresh spinach leaves

- 3 fresh bananas

- 1 inch of fresh ginger

- ½ cup of fresh cilantro

How to Make It:

Begin by washing spinach leaves and cilantro. Peel the lime and remove the seeds from the lime. Wash ginger and cut into pieces. Peel the bananas and then cut them into chunks.

Pour water in the bottom of the blender and then add the spinach leaves and the cilantro. Start blending on low until it turns into a liquid, smooth mixture. Add the lime, bananas and ginger to the blender and start blending again on low. Slowly increase the speed and blend until the smoothie reaches the consistency you want. Makes two servings.

Strawberry and Apple Green Smoothie Recipe

Inspired by a recipe from SparkPeople.com, this recipe combines the flavors of apples and strawberries. It calls for frozen strawberries, since the frozen berries results into a nicely chilled smoothie that is perfect for a warm day. You can always use fresh strawberries and freeze them for a few hours before preparing this green smoothie. It also adds some protein powder to the smoothie, giving a nice protein boost to help you power through your busy day.

What You'll Need:

- 2 tablespoons of flaxseed

- 2 granny smith apples

- 1 cup of fresh spinach leaves

- 1 cup of arugula

- 1 cup of romaine lettuce

- 1 banana

- 2 cups of purified water

- 1 ½ cups of strawberries, frozen

- 1 scoop of your favorite protein powder (not whey protein powder)

How to Make It:

Wash the apples and core them. Cut the apples into chunks. Wash the spinach, arugula and romaine lettuce and sit to the side. Peel the banana and cut it into chunks.

Pour the purified water into the blender. Add the spinach, arugula and romaine on top of the water. Begin blending on low speed. Continue until the greens blend with the water to become smooth. Place the flaxseed, apple chunks, banana chunks, frozen strawberries and protein powder in the blender. Start blending on slow once again, increase the speed as necessary. Continue blending until your smoothie reaches the consistency you prefer. Makes 2-3 servings.

Spinach and Papaya Green Smoothie Recipe

Papaya is known for the antioxidants and beta-carotene that it provides, making it a super healthy fruit. The papaya gives this green smoothie a tropical flare and the lime juice compliments the papaya nicely. The recipe makes a nice 20oz green smoothie that you are sure to enjoy.

What You'll Need:

- 3 cups of chopped spinach leaves, fresh

- 2 cups of sunflower sprouts

- 1 cup of purified water

- 2 limes, juiced

- 2 cups of diced papaya

How to Make It:

Peel the papayas and cut into chunks. Was the spinach and sprouts before using. Juice the limes and reserve the lime juice.

Pour the purified water into your blender, making sure it goes in first. Add sunflower sprouts and spinach leaves to the blender. Begin to blend on low, blending until it becomes a smooth mixture. Take off the lid and add in the diced papaya and the lime juice. Keep blending, increasing the speed until your smoothie is the right consistency. Enjoy and store any leftovers in the refrigerator to enjoy later in the day or the next day. Do not save the smoothie for more than two days.

Orange Juice and Berry Blend Green Smoothie Recipe

The orange juice gives you a large dose of vitamin C and all of the berries provide plenty of important antioxidants as well. This smoothie also includes plenty of potassium and iron, which are both important parts of your diet. If you feel like you are fighting a cold or the flu, try this green smoothie recipe. It should give your immune system a nice boost, helping you fight off sickness.

What You'll Need:

- 1 cup of frozen blueberries

- 1 cup of frozen raspberries

- 2 cups of fresh spinach leaves

- 2 medium bananas

- ¾ cup of freshly squeezed orange juice

- ¾ cup of purified water

How to Make It:

Wash the spinach leaves. Peel the bananas and then cut them into chunks. Squeeze the orange juice from fresh oranges.

Pour the purified water and the orange juice into your blender. Add the spinach leaves and start blending on low. Continue until your mixture is smooth. Open and add the frozen blueberries, frozen raspberries and the chunks of banana. Close the lid and begin blending again. Start slow and then increase the speed. Stop when you reach the consistency that you want for your smoothie. Makes two servings.

Blueberry, Flaxseed and Banana Protein Packed Green Smoothie Recipe

Yummy blueberries, bananas and apples make up a large portion of this fruit packed green smoothie recipe. It also includes a spring salad mix and spinach, making it an excellent detox smoothie to use while you are following the green smoothie detox cleanse. The flaxseed helps to clean out your digestive system and the protein powder will ensure you have the protein you need, whether you are heading to the gym or anticipating a long day working.

What You'll Need:

- 1 large granny smith apple

- 1 cup of spring mix salad greens

- 2 tablespoons of flaxseeds

- ½ cup of red seedless grapes

- 2 cups of fresh spinach leaves

- 1 large banana

- 1 teaspoon of stevia

- 2 cups of purified water

- 1 cup of frozen blueberries

- 1 scoop of hemp or soy protein powder

How to Make It:

Wash the salad greens and the spinach leaves. Wash the apple, core it and then cut it into chunks. Wash the grapes and then peel the banana, cutting the banana into pieces.

Add water, salad greens and spinach to your blender, blending them together until your mixture is smooth. Add the apple chunks, flaxseeds, grapes, banana pieces, stevia, frozen blueberries and protein powder to the blender. Continue blending until you get the smoothie consistency. Add more stevia to taste if desired. Makes 2 servings.

Ginger, Mango and Lemon Green Smoothie Recipe

When your immune system needs a boost, try making this delicious ginger, mango and lemon green smoothie recipe. All the green veggies pack in the nutrients and this is a smoothie that is fairly low in sugars, so it works well for diabetics. The ginger helps to sooth your stomach and also will clear out sinuses, which is an added benefit.

What You'll Need:

- 2 cups of purified water

- 3 cups of mango chunks

- 1 cup of fresh parsley

- 1 lemon

- 1 cup of celery, chopped

- 1 inch of fresh ginger

- 1 cup of fresh spinach leaves

- 1 cucumber, chunked

How to Make It:

Was the parsley, celery, cucumber and spinach leaves.

Cut the celery and cucumber into chunks to make them easier to blend. Peel the lemon and remove its seeds.

Pour the two cups of purified water into the blender. Add the parsley, celery chunks, cucumber chunks and the spinach leaves. Start blending until your mixture becomes smooth. Place the mango chunks, lemon and ginger in the blender. Begin blending again, increasing the blender speed until the mixture is the correct consistency for a smoothie. Makes two servings. Serve immediately and enjoy.

Spinach and Coconut Green Smoothie Recipe

Coconut is full of great nutrients, including important electrolytes and potassium. Coconut water also has lauric acid in it, which helps support thyroid health. Coconut is also wonderful for your skin and helps to make skin look young and beautiful. For this reason, coconut, both the water and the meat, makes a great addition to your green smoothies. This simple recipe, inspired by a recipe from KimberlySnyder.net, only has two ingredients. Enjoy it from time to time as you do the green smoothie cleanse to enjoy all the benefits coconut has to offer.

What You'll Need:

- 3 cups of fresh spinach leaves

- 1 whole coconut

How to Make It:

Wash the spinach and set to the side.

To open the coconut, start by opening it using a cleaver. Pour the water out of the coconut, right into your blender. Then, use a spoon to dig out the coconut meat, adding it to the blender too. Blend the coconut water and coconut meat together until it is smooth.

Add the reserved spinach to the blender. Start blending on low, increasing speed slowly until the mixture becomes smooth. Pour into a glass and enjoy. Makes 1 serving.

Chocolate Cherry and Banana Green Smoothie Recipe

Chocolate covered cherries sound so decadent, and while you are not supposed to have refined sugar on the green smoothie cleanse, this green smoothie will make you feel like you are indulging in chocolate covered cherries. The smoothie includes spinach, so you have the leafy greens you need for the recipe. However, for the delicious sweetness, it combines cacao powder and cherries, giving you a delightful smoothie that tastes almost like a decadent dessert. This is a great smoothie to make when you have a chocolate craving.

What You'll Need:

- 2 cups of fresh cherries, pits removed

- 3 tablespoons of cacao powder

- 2 cups of fresh spinach leaves

- 2 medium bananas

- 2 cups of unsweetened almond milk

- 1 teaspoon of ground cinnamon

How to Make It:

Wash the cherries and remove all the pits. Rinse off the

spinach leaves. Peel bananas and then cut them into pieces.

Pour the unsweetened almond milk into your blender, topping with the spinach leaves. Start blending until the spinach and milk have combined into a smooth mixture. Remove the lid and add the cherries, cacao powder, bananas and ground cinnamon. Place lid back on the blender and start blending once again. Keep blending, increasing the blender speed, until you have a smooth, creamy smoothie. Makes 2 servings. Savor immediately.

Mixed Greens, Mixed Berry and Peach Green Smoothie Recipe

This peachy green smoothie adds mixed berries, apples, mixed greens and flaxseed to the mix. It makes a great green breakfast smoothie because it includes protein powder, which will give you a boost as you start your busy day. If you cannot find fresh peaches, you can always use frozen peaches for this recipe.

What You'll Need:

- 1 granny smith apple

- 2 cups of purified water

- 1 tablespoon of flaxseed

- 1 large peach (or ¾ cup of frozen peaches)

- 1 ½ cups of frozen mixed berries

- 1 cup of fresh spinach leaves

- 1 scoop of hemp or soy protein powder

- 2 teaspoons of stevia

- 2 cups of kale, chopped

How to Make It:

Wash the granny smith apple, core it and then cut it into

chunks. Wash the peach, remove the pit and cut it up. Wash the spinach and kale, chopping the kale into smaller pieces.

Add the purified water to the blender and then add chopped kale and the fresh spinach leaves. Begin blending. Once you have a smooth mixture, stop blending and add the apple chunks, flaxseed, peach pieces, mixed berries, protein powder and stevia. Continue blending until the mixture reaches your desired thickness. Makes 2 large smoothies. Enjoy.

Coconut, Pineapple and Avocado Green Smoothie Recipe

Vitamin E and healthy fats come from the avocado used in this green smoothie. The coconut water helps to regenerate tissue and hydrates your body. The spinach and pineapple offer important nutrients as well. The nutrients found in this smoothie are all great for skin, so continue drinking it regularly if you want to boost your skin health.

What You'll Need:

- 2 cups of fresh coconut water

- 1 ripe avocado

- 2 cups of fresh spinach leaves

- 2 cups of frozen pineapple chunks

How to Make It:

Remove the seed from the avocado and scoop out the flesh. Wash the spinach leaves before using.

Pour the fresh coconut water into the blender and then add your spinach leaves. Turn the blender on low and blend until the spinach and water make a smooth liquid. Add in the avocado and the frozen pineapple. Continue blending, allowing to blend until you have the thickness you desire from your green smoothie. Makes two servings.

Chia Seed Tropical Fruit Green Smoothie Recipe

Inspired by GivemeSomeOven.com, this chia seed tropical fruit green smoothie recipe is sure to please your taste buds. It is packed with fruits and veggies that offer important nutrients for your body. It tastes delightfully sweet as well, which means you will probably be making this recipe more than once. You can have this recipe whipped up in no time for a delicious, nutritious smoothie.

What You'll Need:

- 1 rib of celery

- 3 cups of pineapple, frozen

- 1 tablespoon of chia seeds

- 1 cup of frozen banana slices

- 1 tablespoon of fresh ginger, grated

- ½ lime, juiced

- 3 cups of baby spinach, fresh

How to Make It:

Wash celery and spinach.

Add the lime juice to the bottom of the blender. Place

the spinach in the blender. Blend until smooth and add some purified water if the mixture is too dry. Next, add the celery, pineapple chunks, chia seeds, frozen banana slices and the fresh ginger. Blend again until you have a thick smoothie. If the smoothie is too thick, add some juice or a little water to thin it just a bit. Makes about five cups.

Almond and Berry Blend Green Smoothie Recipe

The almonds in this smoothie give it a nice boost of protein. Protein is important while you are on the green smoothie cleanse because it helps to keep your blood sugar stable, it keeps you feeling full longer and it can help you to avoid cravings as well. The almond milk also adds some protein and makes your smoothie extra creamy and smooth.

What You'll Need:

- 1 medium banana

- 2 cups of fresh spinach leaves

- ½ cup of raw almonds (soaked)

- 2 cups of unsweetened almond milk

- 1 cup of frozen blueberries

- 1 cup of frozen strawberries

How to Make It:

The night before, soak the almonds in water to make them get soft so they can be blended into your smoothie the next day.

Wash the spinach leaves and then peel the banana. Cut the banana into chunks.

Blend together the spinach and the almond milk in the blender until you have a smooth spinach mixture. Once the mixture is smooth, add the banana chunks, almonds, blueberries and strawberries. Start blending again. Continue, increasing the speed of the blender until you have the desired thickness for your delicious green smoothie. Makes two servings.

Ginger, Pineapple and Spirulina Green Smoothie Recipe

The kale and spinach used in this smoothie help to regulate your body's pH and the pineapple includes bromelain, important vitamin C and digestive enzymes. The addition of pineapple also adds sweetness to your smoothie. The added coconut water, cucumber and lemon all help to cleanse your body of toxins.

What You'll Need:

- ½ lemon

- 3 large kale leaves

- 1 teaspoon of spirulina

- 1 cup of spinach leaves

- 1 cup of coconut water

- ½ cucumber

- 1 cup of pineapple, frozen

- 1 inch of ginger, fresh

How to Make It:

Peel the rind off the lemon and remove any seeds. Wash the kale and spinach leaves. Cut the cucumber into chunks and dice up the ginger.

Add the lemon, coconut water, kale leaves and the spinach leaves to your blender, making sure that the water goes on the very bottom. Turn the blender on low and blend until your greens turn into a smooth liquid. Remove the blender lid and add the spirulina, cucumber chunks, pineapple pieces and the slices of ginger. Continue blending until your mixture is smooth and creamy. Makes 1 serving. Enjoy right away.

Orange Cranberry Green Smoothie Recipe

Cranberries are extremely good for you and they pack in a large antioxidant punch. They are a bit tart, but the oranges and bananas in this smoothie will help to balance out the tartness from the cranberries. You are sure to enjoy the combination of the orange and cranberry flavors. This smoothie also offers plenty of fiber and vitamin C, making it a great addition to your green smoothie cleanse plan.

What You'll Need:

- 2 large oranges

- 1 cup of purified water

- 2 large bananas

- 1 cup of fresh cranberries

- 2 cups of fresh kale leaves

How to Make It:

Peel the oranges and pull into sections. Peel the bananas and cut into pieces. Wash the cranberries and the kale leaves before using them in your smoothie.

Add the water and kale leaves to the blender. Start blending on low. Once the mixture is smooth, add in the orange sections, banana pieces and the fresh cranberries. Turn up the speed on your blender, blending until you have the desired thickness for your smoothie. Makes two servings.

NOTE: Freeze the cranberries ahead of time to make the smoothie cold and refreshing.

Basil, Parsley and Blueberry Green Smoothie Recipe

Inspired by a recipe from HealthisHappiness.com, this delicious detoxifying green smoothie includes ingredients that have many health benefits. The cucumbers in it help replenish essential vitamins and the parsley includes important antioxidants and may help prevent cancer. The avocados provide healthy fats for joint and skin health while the basil helps to reduce inflammation in the body while healing the digestive system. Lemon helps to rid the body of toxins and the berries pack in even more antioxidants.

What You'll Need:

- 2 cups of purified water

- 15 leaves of basil

- 1 large banana

- 3-4 ice cubes

- 1 cup of fresh parsley, packed

- ½ cucumber

- ¾ cup of frozen blueberries

- ½ lemon, juiced

- ½ avocado

- Stevia to taste

How to make It:

Wash the basil, parsley and cucumber. Leave the skin on the cucumber and cut into chunks. Peel the banana and then cut into slices. Juice the lemon and set juice to the side. Scoop out the avocado.

Pour the purified water and lemon juice into the blender. Add the basil leaves and the parsley. Start blending on low. Blend until you have a thick, smooth mixture. Add the banana slices, ice cubes, cucumber chunks, frozen blueberries, avocado and stevia to the blender. Start blending again, increasing the speed if necessary. Stop when the smoothie reaches the consistency you desire. Taste and add more stevia to the mixture if you desire. Makes 4.5 cups. Enjoy.

Antioxidant Rich Lime, Mint and Spinach Green Smoothie Recipe

When you want a smoothie packed with antioxidants that will fight off free radicals, you will definitely want to make this smoothie. The cantaloupe includes plenty of vitamin C, vitamin A and beta carotene, all of which help to boost your immune system. Blueberries add more antioxidants, the mint will help to settle the digestive system and you'll enjoy other important nutrients from other healthy ingredients, such as the spinach, lime and apple.

What You'll Need:

- 2 cups of chopped cantaloupe

- ½ lime, juiced

- 1 cup of purified water

- 2 cups of fresh spinach leaves

- 1 granny smith apple

- 1 mint sprig

- ½ cup of frozen blueberries

How to Make It:

Wash the spinach leaves and the mint spring. Remove

the rind from the cantaloupe and cut into chunks. Juice the lime. Core the apple and chop.

Place the water and the fresh spinach leaves into the blender. Start blending the spinach and water on low. Once smooth, add the cantaloupe, lime, apple, mint sprig and frozen blueberries to the blender. Continue blending. Once it comes to the desired thickness, pour into glasses and enjoy. Makes 2 servings.

Chapter 5 – 10 Day Eating Plan

Now that you have a large selection of green smoothie recipes, you are ready to embark on your green smoothie cleanse. However, to make it just a little easier for you, we've put together a 10-day eating plan that you can follow. You don't have to follow this eating plan, but it may prove useful if you lead a busy lifestyle.

Day 1:

Breakfast: Tropical Fruit and Green Leaf Lettuce Green Smoothie

Lunch: Cherry, Blueberry and Raspberry Green Smoothie

Dinner: Sweet Blueberry and Romaine Green Smoothie

Snack: Leftovers from smoothies made throughout the day

Day 2:

Breakfast: Grape, Peach and Coconut Green Smoothie

Lunch: Spicy Cilantro and Romaine Green Smoothie

Dinner: Grapefruit and Kale Green Smoothie

Snack: Leftovers from smoothies made throughout the day

Day 3:

Breakfast: Berry, Kiwi and Avocado Green Smoothie

Lunch: Pina Colada Flavored Spinach and Almond Milk Green Smoothie

Dinner: Baby Lettuce and Pineapple Green Smoothie

Snack: Leftovers from smoothies made throughout the day

Day 4:

Breakfast: Pomegranate, Orange and Banana Green Smoothie

Lunch: Almond Butter and Sweet Red Grape Green Smoothie

Dinner: Romaine and Banana Green Smoothie

Snack: Leftovers from smoothies made throughout the day

Day 5:

Breakfast: Peach and Spinach Green Smoothie

Lunch: Coconut, Almond and Cantaloupe Green Smoothie

Dinner: Flaxseed Berry Blend Green Smoothie

Snack: Leftovers from smoothies made throughout the day

Day 6:

Breakfast: Romaine, Strawberry and Grape Green Smoothie

Lunch: Pear, Apple and Banana Green Smoothie

Dinner: Mango, Banana and Spinach Green Smoothie

Snack: Leftovers from smoothies made throughout the day

Day 7:

Breakfast: Protein Powder and Chia Seed Green Smoothie

Lunch: Mango, Pineapple and Cilantro Green Smoothie

Dinner: Spinach and Papaya Green Smoothie

Snack: Leftovers from smoothies made throughout the day

Day 8:

Breakfast: Blueberry, Flaxseed and Banana Protein Packed Green Smoothie

Lunch: Ginger Cilantro Limeade Green Smoothie

Dinner: Spinach and Coconut Green Smoothie

Snack: Leftovers from smoothies made throughout the day

Day 9:

Breakfast: Strawberry and Apple Green Smoothie

Lunch: Mixed Greens, Mixed Berry and Peach Green Smoothie

Dinner: Ginger, Mango and Lemon Green Smoothie

Snack: Leftovers from smoothies made throughout the day

Day 10:

Breakfast: Orange Juice and Berry Blend Green Smoothie

Lunch: Chocolate Cherry and Banana Green Smoothie

Dinner: Chia Seed Tropical Fruit Green Smoothie

Snack: Leftovers from smoothies made throughout the day

Conclusion:

After following the green smoothie diet for 10 days, you need to be prepared to break the cleanse correctly. Since you have been only eating liquids, you need to slowly go back to eating whole foods. Plan on taking 3-4 days to start adding whole foods back into your diet. Keep drinking smoothies during the day and gradually start adding more solid foods to your diet, such as salads, sautéed veggies or other foods that are easy on your body. Make sure your diet is very light for the first few days. You can start by doing smoothies for two meals and eating one light meal. After three days, eat two meals and have a smoothie for one meal. However, if you want to enjoy the best results from your cleanse, make sure you eat healthy foods as you introduce whole foods into your diet. If you start eating foods that are bad for you, you'll end up in the same place you were before the cleanse.

To keep losing weight, try replacing one meal a day with a green smoothie. This will help you keep getting important nutrients while encouraging weight loss. If you have a significant amount of weight to lose, you could have smoothies for two of your meals and go with one, light, healthy meal each day.

Since you want to keep your weight loss going, keep using the green smoothie recipes in this book, even after you finish the initial 10-day cleanse. You will continue to reap all the benefits smoothies have to offer and changing your lifestyle will result in weight loss and a healthier body.

CPSIA information can be obtained
at www.ICGtesting.com
Printed in the USA
LVOW04s1623091215

466131LV00022B/1307/P

9 781633 834675